Seattle 4.16.10

# vegan in 30 days
Get healthy. Save the world.

## sarah taylor

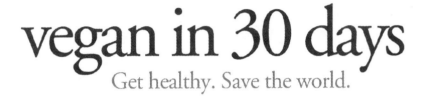

# vegan in 30 days

Get healthy. Save the world.

## sarah taylor

# vegan success stories

*"Adopting a very high nutrient vegan lifestyle allowed me to lose 26 pounds in just 6 weeks, lowered my systolic blood pressure by 25 points, and also increased my energy tremendously... I am never going back!"*

~ **Maarten V.** - Voorschoten, The Netherlands

*"I didn't become vegan for health reasons, but found, nonetheless, that I have much more energy and I never feel sluggish after eating!"*

~ **Elliot G.** - Tacoma, WA

*"Since becoming a vegan, I lost about 10 pounds and lowered my cholesterol by 107 points! While the health aspect is fantastic, it is my love of animals that keeps me vegan. My conscience is clear and I feel good about the example I set for others, even if they do not follow my path."*

~ **Corrine W.** - Newington CT

*"The first few weeks are the hardest; everyone thinks you're crazy, and it seems like everything is made with eggs and dairy. But soon you start feeling more energetic, thinner, and better than ever, which makes it all worthwhile!"*

~ **Andrea B.** - Woodinville, WA

*"A little over a year ago I was on Lipitor with a cholesterol level of 234, and was about 25 pounds overweight. I was also on allergy and nasal medications and had the beginning stages of arthritis in my fingers. After adopting a vegan diet, my cholesterol has dropped to 160, my allergies are gone, the arthritis is no longer an issue, I've lost over 25 pounds and was able to eliminate the usage of all medication. I have much more energy and feel consistently better now. My husband also joined me and at 6'6 was close to 250 pounds with a cholesterol level of 199. After adopting a vegan lifestyle, he lost 45 pounds and dropped his cholesterol to 158. Both of us just turned 60, and wish we would have adopted this non-processed, vegan way of eating long ago."*

~ **Kathy E.** - Scottsdale, AZ

*"Since I gave up eating any 'creatures great or small' I feel much younger than my passport says. I like the idea that I'm not eating anyone's mother too!"*

~ **Virginia K.** - Gig Harbor, WA

*"The one thing I was most unaware of and surprised about when I first learned about vegetarianism was that humans have no nutritional need for animal products, and that plant-based foods are nutritionally superior. Like most of us, I had assumed that animal products were necessary for our health. How else could one justify the needless suffering that animals are put through to become our food? The fact is that it cannot, and becoming a vegetarian and ultimately a vegan became mandatory."*

~ **Ron S.** - San Francisco, CA

*"Going vegan helped me feel less guilty about my food choices, better about my body, and helped me recover from an eating disorder."*

~ **Sarah K.** - San Antonio, TX

"My pregnancy was stellar because of my vegan diet. I had no morning sickness, I was so comfortable, and I felt great. My newborn was super-healthy. She hasn't had an ear infection yet, and when she gets a cold, she kicks it very quickly. I'm sure that's because she never had dairy, and doesn't have a build up of mucus."

~ **Sarah G.** - Santa Cruz, CA

"Since becoming a vegan the intestinal problems that I dealt with for the first 42 years of my life disappeared."

~ **Ann W.** - Belvedere, CA

"Since becoming vegans, my husband and I have virtually eliminated any chance of experiencing the vascular/heart disease so prevalent in our families. Our lipid figures indicate that we will never need the quadruple coronary bypass surgeries required by both our fathers. Just as important to me, I now maintain my ideal weight of 110 with a way of eating that I love and can cheerfully live with forever. I had been a yo-yo dieter for over thirty years, with a top weight of 165."

~ **Laurie M.** - Norman, OK

*"After shifting to a plant-based diet for health reasons in 2003, I soon learned about many other reasons that supported my decision. World Hunger: On the amount of land required to feed 100 people the rich western diet, you can feed 2,000 plant-eaters. Environment: According to a 2006 U.N. Report, raising livestock for human consumption causes 30% more global warming than ALL transportation in the world... combined. Further, to produce just ten pounds of steak requires the same amount of water required for ALL household uses for a family of four for a FULL year. Finally: Not only do we destroy our environment and torture billions of animals a year to feed our very unhealthy craving for animal foods, but we have created an unsustainable system that simply must change for the future of life on Planet Earth... for our children who follow us."*

~ **Jim H.** - Stonington, CT

*"Ever since I adopted a nutrient dense, plant-based eating style I am a changed woman. I have accomplished so much, have so much more energy and a whole new outlook on life. I've lost 76 pounds so far too!"*

~ **Isabel P.** - Ontario, Canada

*"When we learned that if people cut back on animal consumption by just 10%, it would save enough grain to feed the world's hungry, we became vegan overnight. We felt we couldn't call ourselves environmentalists and continue to eat anything but a plant-based diet."*

~ **Sheila H. and Spencer B.** - Seattle, WA

*"Although initially my journey to better health seemed only an easy way to lose weight (just eat tons of veggies!), as I continued educating myself I could no longer deny that the benefits of eating healthfully were so much greater than just losing a few pounds. I began to see this as a gift I could give my children and so far, so good. My 2 1/2 year old is one of the few toddlers I know who heartily gobbles down eggplant, broccoli, and artichokes. We all do so much to protect our children, be it car seats, bike helmets or teaching them the dangers of smoking. In my mind, teaching them to eat vegan is yet another way to keep them healthy and safe."*

~ **Colleen E.** - Springfield, VA

*"I'm 45 and in menopause—my symptoms are much less than my friends. I'm sure it's because I don't eat dairy."*

~ **Sarah G.** - Santa Cruz, CA

*"One of the most positive changes our family has made in the past two years was deciding eat vegan. My 'meat and potatoes' Iowa-raised husband took to it easier than I ever would have imagined. He not only lowered his weight by 40 pounds in 5 months, but he was also able to stop taking Lipitor, as his cholesterol dropped by over 100 points. He also had to get a new contact lens prescription as his eyesight improved. I was able to lose 65 pounds in 7 months and have never felt better... the increased energy and healthy hair and nails are just a few visual results. I always think about the benefits we can't see, that are taking place inside our bodies... leading us down a road to a healthy life, free from many of the diseases of western culture. And the importance of showing our two boys, ages 6 and 9, how everything they eat impacts their future is of vital relevance as the number of sick and obese children is reaching unprecedented levels. I just wish that this lifestyle was more openly embraced by mainstream society."*

~ **Robyn R.** - Glendale, AZ

*"Many people think vegans are too skinny. Interestingly, I was actually underweight before going vegan, and the vegan diet helped me to put on five needed pounds. I think the vegan diet helps you achieve and maintain a healthy weight—whether that means you need to gain or lose weight."*

~ **Elliot G.** - Tacoma, WA

*"Although I'd been a vegetarian for 12 years, I made the leap to a vegan diet three years ago. It wasn't really that difficult (yes, you CAN get all the protein you need from beans and soy) and I'm amazed at how much better I feel. I haven't gotten sick—not even with a common cold—in three years!"*

~ **Andrea B.** - Woodinville, WA

---

For every person who continually
strives to do things better,
and do better things.

———————— 🍎 ————————

# table of contents

# acknowledgments

I'd like to begin by expressing my sincere thanks to my husband, Mark, who encourages me to follow my dreams. You are the love of my life, and I am blessed to have found you!

I'd like to thank the many vegan authors and speakers who have profoundly changed my life, including, but not limited to: John Robbins, Joel Fuhrman, MD, Colin Campbell, PhD, Caldwell Esselstyn, MD, Neal Barnard, MD, Erik Marcus, and Gail Eisnitz.

I'd like to thank my family, my MasterMind group, my business partners and my friends for their encouragement, advice, and support. Most especially: George and Virginia Kenefick, Karen Kenefick-Massand, Norm Ferguson, Sandra Kolb, Peter Stankovich, Sharon Galbraith, Carol Schaeffer, Charlotte Cavoores, Holly King, Ken Smith, Dick Bownes, Tamra Woodman, Rebecca James, and Joel Fuhrman, MD.

Special thanks to the people who contributed to the physical creation of this book: Robyn Rolfes at Creative Syndicate, Inc, Melody Morris at Central Plains Book, a division of Sun Graphics LLC, and Sharon Galbraith, Editor.

Finally, my thanks and amazement to Lorri Bauston, Frank Allen, and others who are saving the world. You do good work!

# introduction

So, you want to go vegan! You're not alone: People are turning to veganism in record numbers, for a variety of reasons: the promise of a thin body, a goal of better health, to prevent or reverse disease, a desire to radically decrease one's carbon footprint on the environment, a hope of feeding more people on the planet, and outrage over the suffering that animals must endure to become our food.

There are many reasons you may want to try the vegan diet. **The purpose of this book is not to convince you to go vegan—it is to help you take the steps to do it successfully and healthfully.** I am assuming that you picked up this book because you've already found a reason to go vegan; therefore, you will not find a lot of arguments in the following pages for why you should eat this way, but you *will* find solid, well-researched advice on how to do it healthfully and successfully.

So, as you read this book, there are some things I'd like you to keep in mind:

- First, I want to emphasize that my goal is for you to adopt a healthy vegan diet by the end of 30 days. We all have varying ideas of what is healthy, and I must admit that mine are pretty strict compared to the average American's standards, but I feel a duty to ensure that I don't lead you down the road of the "junk food vegan." Therefore, you'll notice a strong emphasis on health throughout the book, and some of my suggestions are related to general health, not just the vegan diet.

- Second, as a vegan, you will obviously not be eating animal products by the end of this program. If you have large dollar volumes of animal foods in your kitchen right now, start using them up, or plan to donate them or give them away to friends or family. You can look through the Table of Contents to see on which days you will be eliminating which non-vegan foods, and plan accordingly.

- Third, these 30 steps are carefully designed and are time tested. While you may be tempted to skip a step or two, resist that temptation—the step you skip just might be the most important one for your long-term success!

- Fourth, some of my steps involve investing some money. You'll need some books, new foods for your pantry, a new cooking gadget or two, and if you're overweight, you'll quite possibly need some new clothes! If money is scarce for you, simply be creative. Instead of buying a book, borrow it from the library; instead of buying a new high-end cooking gadget, buy a used, lower-end one. In fact, when you buy used items, you'll not only save money, but you'll help save the environment by recycling someone else's used product! You're smart… be resourceful!

- Fifth, take your time and be kind to yourself. Don't demand perfection from yourself. Adopting a vegan diet can be challenging, so if you need more than 30 days to do this program, that's perfectly fine! You may find that one of the steps could take you a few weeks, while a few other steps can be done on the same day. The important thing to ensure your success is to be working on a step every single day. Don't let a day go by when you aren't working on your current step. Make that a commitment. Remember, it's much better to be successful over the long term— even if it means taking longer than 30 days to complete the program—than to try to rush steps when you're not ready, and end up failing.

- Sixth and finally, I'd like to make a comment about detoxification. When you change from an unhealthy diet to a healthy one in a short period of time, it is common to have detoxification symptoms as your body rids itself of toxins. Detox symptoms generally last from a few days to a few weeks, and could include symptoms such as:

  - Headaches
  - Fatigue
  - Nausea
  - Runny nose
  - Light-headedness
  - Dizziness
  - Minor aches and pains
  - Excessive sweating
  - Other symptoms

  Because you are embarking on a 30 day step-by-step plan, rather than going "cold turkey," you may not experience many of these symptoms, if any at all. Whether you experience detoxification symptoms or not will depend on the level toxins currently in your body, how much difference there is between the vegan diet and your current diet, as well as how sensitive your body is to change. If your body is sensitive to change, you may want to take at least two or three days for each of the 30 steps.

If you experience any of the above symptoms, do two things: First, consider calling your physician, if you feel more than a little discomfort. However, try to avoid medicating the symptoms if at all possible—it's important for you to "hear" what your body is telling you, and you'll only know you've made it through detox if the symptoms naturally go away on their own, without medication. Second, celebrate! Don't reach for ice cream or cake to celebrate, but have a happy mental celebration, knowing that your body is ridding itself of toxins. Once your body has cleaned out these toxins, you will feel fantastic, and have tons of energy.

I am very glad you're here, and honored that you've invested in this book. Now, sit back, and start reading. This may very well be the first day of a brand new life!

# DAY

# 1

## why do you want to be vegan?

The first—and probably the most important—step of any goal is to know why you want to achieve it. Many people set goals that they never reach, and often it's because they haven't given themselves a compelling enough reason to go to the effort and make the sacrifices they need to reach the goal.

As a general rule of thumb, the bigger the goal, the better the reason you'll need to convince yourself to stick with it. I find it amazing how, whenever I wanted to lose weight in the past, I'd really want it so that I'd look better; however, as soon as a jumbo chocolate chip cookie found it's way in front of me, I seemed to forget why I was even on a diet! Apparently, vanity was not a big enough reason for me to stick with this goal—which is why I always made excuses to justify cheating. Excuses, tied to a poor reason for achieving your goal, always leads to failure.

Interestingly, in my quest to lose weight, I came across a book that discussed the very sad conditions of the animals in slaughterhouses and factory farms. Being a bona-fide animal lover, I was extremely disturbed by what I read, and instantly went vegan—losing all the weight as a welcomed side effect. In the end, it wasn't a vain desire to lose weight that helped me to finally lose it—it was a desire to be kinder to animals.

Your objective today is to examine why it is that you want to be a vegan in 30 days. Is your reason compelling enough so that you will stick with it for 30 days? What about your whole life, if that's your ultimate goal?

If you are having trouble coming up with a compelling enough reason to go vegan, start to think about what your life might be like in 5 years if you don't make any changes now. For many people, imagining things being exactly the same as they are today—or likely far worse—is a very compelling reason to instigate change! Another option is to read about veganism—there are some extremely persuasive arguments that you simply may not have uncovered yet. You can skip to Day 10 and read Diet for a New America, the book that prompted me to go vegan, if you feel you need some more influential reasons.

## assignment

Becoming vegan is a big goal. Find a big reason for why you want it. Right down your reason(s), either in a paragraph or in a list, and put it somewhere you will read it every day. Use compelling language, so that every time you read it, you are reinvigorated toward your goal.

The best lists or paragraphs are detailed: instead of just writing "I want to be vegan so I can beat diabetes," write down all the things you'll be able to do when you achieve your goal. For example, "I want to be vegan so I can beat diabetes. Once I am no longer obese and reliant on medications, I'll be able to play with my kids in the yard for hours, I'll finally feel proud of myself, I won't worry about going blind or losing a limb from advanced diabetes, I'll buy a sexy black dress and go dancing..." You may even want to cut some pictures out of a magazine that show the person you want to become. If you can picture your life once you've reached your goal, that vision will be very motivational to you!

**tip**

You should never need to feel hungry—or guilty—on a vegan diet. Eat as many fruits and veggies as you want, all day long, and feel terrific for making such healthy choices!

# DAY

# 2

## know the basics

Many people are confused about what a vegan diet actually is. Some people mistakenly think it's the same as a vegetarian diet, or that it includes fish or poultry. Here is the real definition of the vegan diet:

**A vegan diet is one that does not include any flesh from animals, or any animal products.**

This essentially means no meat, poultry, fish, dairy products or eggs. Instead, vegans eat foods that come straight from nature's garden—lots of fresh, crisp and colorful fruits and vegetables, beans, grains, nuts and seeds. It is a plant-based diet.

Sometimes, when people who are interested in switching to a vegan diet realize just how many non-vegan ingredients they are consuming, they feel overwhelmed. The best strategy for dealing with this is exactly what you are doing with this book: simply tackle the diet in steps. For example, instead of trying to give up all non-vegan items at once, you can start by giving up red meat, and eat poultry and fish instead. Once you're perfectly comfortable without red meat, you can then give up poultry and just eat fish. At the same time, you can decrease the amount of meat and dairy on your plate, and increase the amount of beans, grains and veggies.

If the idea of giving up all flesh leaves you worried, take comfort: Most people find that what gives meat the flavor they enjoy is not the meat itself, but the sauces and spices they put on the meat. Eventually, you'll feel comfortable putting those sauces and spices over veggies or pasta instead, and eliminating all meat, poultry and fish from your diet altogether.

Once you've eliminated the "biggies" from your diet, like meat and dairy, you'll work on giving up other products, like whey, gelatin, and lecithin. We'll get to these less familiar products on Day 28. My experience is that this step-by-step approach is the most successful way to become a true, lasting vegan.

Since good health is so vital to our well-being, I'd like to make a note here about "junk food vegans," and how to eat a healthy vegan diet. The vegan diet is naturally very, very healthful. Focusing on veggies, fruits, beans, grains, nuts and seeds, it is truly nature's diet. However, with the rising popularity of the vegan diet, vegan "junk food" is becoming more and more commonplace. These foods are numerous, and include items like baked goods that use margarine in place of butter, and soy ice cream made with loads of sugar. They may be vegan, but they're not necessarily healthful.

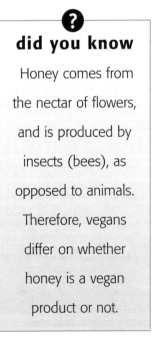

**did you know**

Honey comes from the nectar of flowers, and is produced by insects (bees), as opposed to animals. Therefore, vegans differ on whether honey is a vegan product or not.

Any food that has high amounts of salt, sugar or fat—whether that food is vegan or not—is simply not healthy for you. Processed foods are almost guaranteed to have too much of at least one of these ingredients, if not all three, and so I believe that one of the best things you can do for your overall health is to avoid eating too many foods that come from boxes, cans or jars—these are generally processed and/or include unnecessary ingredients like added salt or sugar. Even non-processed foods can still be unhealthy—like the vegan cookies at my local bakery whose main ingredients are margarine, oil and sugar. I'm not saying you should never eat these items, but for the sake of your health, make sure it's not a daily event.

> **tip**
>
> If you buy your produce from local farmers, it will have far fewer miles to travel to get to your kitchen, leaving a much smaller carbon footprint on the world. Buying grapes from Chile, when you live in Boston, is not an environmentally friendly choice!

For your health, I encourage you to buy as much of your produce as you can from organic growers. You will be buying a lot of produce once you go vegan, and scientists have shown links between cancer and many of the herbicides, pesticides and fertilizers that are sprayed on non-organic foods. While the government will tell you that the amounts used are not harmful, many independent scientists disagree. It's simply not worth the risk. Plus, organic, in-season produce tastes so much better than conventional produce!

Finally, there has been a lot of emphasis on carbohydrates in recent years, as low-carb diets gained popularity. For vegans, much of the diet is made of carbohydrates, but most of them are healthy carbohydrates that are found in fruits, veggies, beans and grains. It should be noted that refined grain products like white bread, white rice and most baked goods cause your body's glucose levels to spike, while complex carbohydrates like those found in brown rice and 100% whole grains and breads, are actually very healthy for you, and don't cause the same glucose spike.

For your health, always aim for 100% whole grain products, and avoid salt, sugar and fat as much as possible. Although it's very rare, even a vegan can become unhealthy and even overweight. Since you are committing to a new way of eating, make sure you commit to doing it healthfully!

## assignment
Get online and research the vegan diet. Devote at least 30 minutes to learning about how different people define it, and what products are on the market that are vegan and not vegan.

# DAY

# 3

## fruit and veg cleanse

Today you will start your journey with a 24-hour fruit and vegetable cleanse. Ideally, you will eat only organic raw fruits and veggies in their whole, natural form. If you must, you can make a hot dish, as long as all the ingredients are fresh fruits and veggies. Avoid anything canned, jarred or frozen, as salt or sugary syrups are often added.

Go through your grocer's produce section, and select foods that tempt you. Perhaps you'll go home and make a huge salad with bell peppers, cucumbers, corn, carrots, green onion, sprouts and avocado. You can use a vinaigrette or nut-based dressing on your salad. Maybe you'll have a large bowl of cut melon and berries. You decide. You might choose to create a cooked dish, such as ratatouille or potato and pea curry using low-sodium vegetable broth, but try to stick as closely to 100% raw, organic fruits and vegetables as you can.

If you feel hungry, don't panic—just eat more! Foods that are high in protein and fat, like steak, have a very long transit time in our intestines, because it takes our bodies a long time to break them down and process them. This gives us a very full feeling, often lulling us to sleep, as blood rushes to our gut to digest the food. Fruits and vegetables, on the other hand, have the shortest transit times of all foods; you should never feel like you need a nap after a meal of fruits and veggies. Because they clear our system relatively quickly, they naturally leave us feeling hungry sooner than if we'd had a steak. Don't feel guilty about feeling hungry! Simply make another salad, or bite into an apple. As I see it, one of the great benefits of being vegan is that I can guiltlessly eat all day, and maintain a slender weight!

## assignment
Eat only whole fruits and vegetables today, preferably raw, organic, and fresh from your grocer's produce section. Small amounts of condiments, like vinaigrette dressing, can be used to supplement your food.

# DAY
# 4

## eliminate red meat

You've committed to going vegan, and today is the day that you will take the first major step toward becoming vegan. Starting today, you will eliminate all red meat from your diet and your kitchen. As you know, vegans don't eat meat, poultry, fish, dairy products or eggs, and you will be eliminating one of these items every four days until the end of the 30-day program.

The first step for most vegetarians and vegans is to give up "meat." I put the word meat in quotes, because it seems that there are many different definitions of it. I believe that anything with flesh—including fish—is meat. However, I understand that many people separate poultry and fish from "meat." For today, the definition of meat includes what most people would call "red meat:" beef, pork, lamb, venison and any other flesh food that is not fish or fowl.

Giving up meat is probably much easier than you'd imagine. Instead of a hamburger, you can have a chicken burger; instead of a steak, you can have salmon. There are so many options available at any grocery aisle or restaurant, that there are bound to be plenty of choices that will sound good to you and don't include meat.

If you are saying to yourself, "But my favorite meal in the entire world is a cheeseburger! Nothing else will ever do!" then let me kindly point out a stark fact: Almost every vegan had to give up his or her favorite food to become vegan. The good news is that there is almost always a great vegan substitute for your favorite food. If you love cheeseburgers, you can have a veggie burger; if you love ice cream, you can have soy ice cream; if you love chocolate, you can have dark chocolate. As a self-proclaimed macaroni and cheese lover, I can honestly say that the best macaroni and cheese I've ever had in my life (vegan or not) comes from a 100% vegan restaurant in Tacoma, Washington. Sometimes the substitutes are as good as, or better than, the original food, sometimes they're close enough to make do, and sometimes, unfortunately, they just don't make the grade. Tomorrow you will be learning all about substitute foods, so don't worry—no matter what your favorite foods are right now, you will likely find a great replacement.

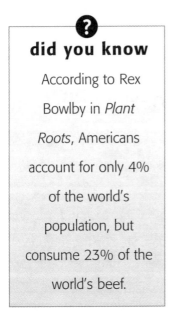

**did you know**

According to Rex Bowlby in *Plant Roots*, Americans account for only 4% of the world's population, but consume 23% of the world's beef.

However, even if you never find a suitable replacement for your favorite food, I'm betting that you won't mind a bit at the end of 30 days. Here's why (and it's the BIG secret to succeeding on the vegan diet): Once you have really cleansed your palate by eating a healthy vegan diet— avoiding animals, animal products, added salt, sugar and fats—for 30 days, your taste buds revert back to their original state—just like they were when you were a baby. This means that an apple will explode on

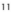

your tongue, and corn will taste better than a cheeseburger ever did. I know this sounds impossible, but if you really eat a clean vegan diet for about 30 days, you will come to see that this is absolutely true. Since you won't be 100% vegan until day 28 of this plan, you may need to continue on for another 3-4 weeks to achieve these results. After this time, you'll bite into an apple one day and be amazed at just how good it tastes! Many people who eat a truly healthy vegan diet report having cravings for kale and other leafy green veggies! So once again...

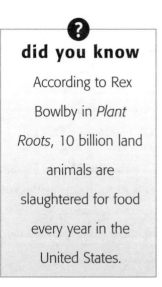

**did you know**

According to Rex Bowlby in *Plant Roots*, 10 billion land animals are slaughtered for food every year in the United States.

## The big secret to succeeding on the vegan diet:

**When you eat a healthy vegan diet—avoiding animals, animal products, and added salt, sugar and fats—your cravings for unhealthy food will disappear, and your taste buds will become hypersensitive, making raw fruits and vegetables taste delectable!**

Since you had a fruit and veg cleanse yesterday, you're on your way toward this new state of well-being. Eliminating meat will take you once step closer!

# assignment

Eliminate all meat from your diet and your kitchen. Remove meat from your refrigerator, freezer and cupboards. If there are other people in your household who are not going vegan, make specific areas in your fridge, freezer and cupboards for their meat products, and keep your food separate.

Donate any of your remaining meat to a local food bank—they will be thrilled for the unusual windfall!

# DAY
# 5

## find substitutes

Many people wonder how someone can stick to a vegan diet. It seems so strict to most people, and they wonder how we can live without America's favorite foods like ice cream and cheeseburgers. However, we vegans know a little secret: for every tasty animal product on the market, there is *almost always* an equivalent vegan substitute! Do you miss your sordid affair with Ben & Jerry? No problem, try one of the incredible soy ice creams on the market. Dying for some mac & cheese? Get the *Un-Cheese Cookbook* by Joanne Stepaniak and create your own. Dying for sausage and eggs for breakfast? Try the soy sausage on the market, and make some scrambled tofu. You'll be shocked by how good most of the substitutes are! Even my seriously carnivorous dad loves my bean chili with cilantro pesto, and I never make my veggie ceviche without getting a request for the recipe.

Since many people are becoming vegetarian and vegan, the substitute products are getting better and are more widely available. However, I will give a caveat here: You *must* be patient and try several brands. A perfect example is with soy milk. The first time I tried soymilk, I swore off it forever - the brand I tried was horrible! However, someone told me to try other brands, and said she particularly liked the Westsoy brand. I tried it, and couldn't tell the difference between it and the cow's milk I used to drink! So, promise yourself that you'll try several brands of each item if you need to. It's actually quite fun! But remember, there will still be times when you'll come across a horrible box of vegan cookies or soy cheese.

There is one other note I'd like to make: I've already mentioned that, while it's quite rare, vegans can certainly be unhealthy. Therefore, I want to be clear that, while I think substitute foods can be great in helping you transition to a vegan diet, many of them are filled with salt, sugar and even fat, so I do not suggest that you eat a lot of substitute foods. However, if you are currently eating the

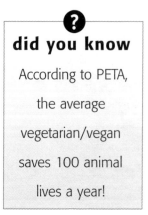

**did you know**

According to PETA, the average vegetarian/vegan saves 100 animal lives a year!

standard American diet filled with meat, dairy and fried foods, these substitutes can really help you transition into a much more healthful vegan diet. Just like you shouldn't eat Ben & Jerry's every day, you shouldn't eat soy ice cream every day either; while it's a much healthier option, it's still not ideal. However, substitutes are great transition items, and are also great for when you're an established, healthy vegan, but just need an occasional treat!

OK, one more note: I told you about the "big vegan secret" in the last chapter - once you have really cleansed your palate by eating a healthful vegan diet for 30 days, you'll lose your cravings for unhealthy food, and your taste buds revert back to their original state; that's when natural fruits and veggies will start tasting unbelievable. However, if you eat salty or sugary substitute foods—and substitute foods are often filled with salt and sugar—you won't be able to achieve a cleansed palate... another reason to only use them sparingly!

Consult the table on page 17 to help you find substitutes and make transitions as you adopt a vegan diet. When you are new to the vegan diet, it's alright to eat a lot of foods from the middle column, but eventually, you'll want to eat most of your food from the far right column, in addition to lots of fruits and vegetables.

## assignment
Go to the local health food store or the health food aisle in your local supermarket. Look for soy-based meat, cheese, and dairy substitutes. If someone is shopping in the same aisles, you may want to ask if they have any experience with the products, and what brands they recommend. Buy at least one new substitute product that you have not tried before.

| OLD CHOICE | SUBSTITUTE CHOICE | BEST CHOICE |
|---|---|---|
| Meat (Beef, Pork, Turkey, Chicken, Fish) | Tofu, Tempeh or Seitan. Soy versions of Sausage, Pepperoni, Burgers and Ground Beef. | Beans |
| Cheese | Vegan Cheese (avoid the ingredient casein) | Nutritional Yeast (as an ingredient, not a topping) |
| Yogurt or Sour Cream | Vegan Yogurt or Sour Cream (avoid the ingredient casein) | Omit |
| Creamy Salad Dressings and Dips | Vinaigrette Dressings, Hummus, Baba Ganoush | Vinegar, Lemon Juice, No-Oil Hummus, Nut-based Dressings |
| Potato Chips | Baked Tortilla Chips and Salsa | Veggies with Salsa or Hummus |
| Bread | Bread made without Eggs, Milk or Butter | Sprouted or 100% Whole Grain Bread with no Eggs or Butter |
| Butter | Oil (or rarely, Margarine) | Water (for Sautéing Vegetables) |
| Eggs | Scrambled Tofu; EnerG Egg Replacer, Applesauce or Bananas for Baking | EnerG Egg Replacer, Applesauce or Bananas for Baking |
| Milk | Soymilk, Rice Milk, Nut Milk | Soymilk, Rice Milk, Nut Milk |
| Chocolate | Dark Chocolate | Fruit |
| Ice Cream | Soy Ice Cream, Sorbet | Fruit |

# DAY
# 6

## get a beautiful fruit bowl, and keep it filled!

In his often-quoted book, Mindless Eating, author Brian Wansink reports that one of the biggest predictors of what and how much you will eat is determined by what food is in closest proximity to you. This shouldn't surprise anyone—it's the candy bowl phenomenon: You will eat more candy at work if a colleague has a candy bowl on her desk, and the closer she sits to you, the more you will eat.

Knowing this, wouldn't it be better—if you were prone to grazing—to pick up a piece of fruit instead of something much less healthy? To avoid slipping back into non-vegan foods, or eating too much vegan junk food, stock your refrigerator with lots of freshly cut veggies for salads and dipping into hummus, and have a fruit bowl on your dining table filled with gorgeous, ripe fruits. Do not keep vegan junk food in the house… if you want it that badly, you can go out and buy it. At work and when traveling, always carry some raw nuts or easy-to-eat fruit with you in case you get hungry.

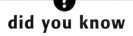

## did you know

According to a 2006 United Nations Food & Agricultural report, the international meat industry generates roughly 18% of the world's greenhouse gas emissions—even more than transportation.

## assignment

If you don't already have one, buy a gorgeous fruit bowl that you just love seeing on your dining table or in your kitchen. (You can find some great bargains at thrift stores!) Then fill it with your favorite fruits—and keep it filled!

# DAY
# 7

## start each day with a green smoothie

Have you ever heard that you're supposed to chew your food 50 times before you swallow it? The reason for that advice is that vital nutrients inside the food we eat are often contained within thick cell walls. Those nutrients can't be released unless the cell walls are broken up adequately. The cell walls are broken up, as you can guess, when we chew our food.

However, if you're like me, you don't always chew—you inhale! As many times as I've heard the advice to chew thoroughly, I only remember to do it for the first few mouthfuls of my meal, and then I completely forget. Not to worry—there's another way to break those nutrients out of the cell walls, and it's even more efficient that chewing! The process is simply blending your food.

> **tip**
>
> Spinach and Romaine lettuce have the least flavor of all the dark leafy greens, making them ideal for your green smoothies.

Obviously, we wouldn't enjoy our food if everything we ate was blended up like baby food. However, there are several foods that do work very well blended, that you can incorporate into your daily routines.

One of the tastiest and most nutrient-packed meals you can make with your blender is a green smoothie. Green smoothies get their green color from spinach or other dark leafy greens you put into them, which are the most nutrient-rich foods on earth. Surprisingly, as their rising popularity suggests, they taste great! Here's why: You can make a green smoothie by simply adding greens to your otherwise all-fruit smoothie. You probably won't taste them at all—they'll simply turn your smoothie green. If you like strawberry-banana smoothies, for example, you'll still love them with the greens thrown in!

My favorite green smoothie is easy to make, truly delicious, and incredibly healthful. I simply take a bag of frozen tropical fruit, add a couple of cups of water to cover the blades of the blender, and two handfuls of spinach. Everyone agrees it's delicious, and it's only about 300 calories for 32 ounces! Best yet, it's got more nutrition in it than most Americans get in a full day of eating fried and packaged foods.

Some hints for making green smoothies:

- I highly recommend a Vitamix brand blender. Over time, the motors on most regular blenders' engines will burn out trying to blend ice or frozen items. However, a Vitamix is made to do this. It is often described as a blender on steroids. If you can afford to buy one (or get one used on the internet) I highly recommend it.

- If you use a cup or two of hot water to make your smoothie, it will bring the temperature of your smoothie up just enough to help ward off ice-cream headaches.

- Make sure you buy frozen fruit that has nothing added to it—no sugar, no syrups, no juices—only 100% whole fruit, preferably organic.

- Berries are some of the most nutritious fruits available, so try a berry-blend smoothie.

- If you you're nervous about adding greens to a perfectly good fruit smoothie, try adding a few leaves, and see if you can taste a difference. Then add a few more. Eventually, you'll realize that you can add one or two large handfuls of spinach leaves without even tasting it.

## assignment

Make a green smoothie for breakfast, lunch or a snack today. Commit to having one green smoothie a day for the next seven days. It will become a habit you won't ever want to give up!

---

### tip

Soups are another great item to blend. If you create a pot of soup and blend about a 1/3 of it, you have just created a creamy consistency without adding cream!

---

# DAY
# 8

## eliminate poultry

Starting today, you will eliminate all poultry from your diet and your kitchen, including chicken, turkey and other fowl. For me, this was the biggest *mental* hurdle, but surprisingly, it was the easiest *physical* hurdle. It was the biggest mental hurdle because I had not eaten red meat for some time, so chicken and fish were the only animal flesh I ate. I didn't know how to cook fish at the time (or much else, for that matter!) but I knew how to cook chicken. My signature dish was Parmesan chicken… if I gave up chicken, what would I make? Plus, there were a lot of chicken dishes I really liked.

**tip**

Salt is included in so many foods you buy. Start eliminating it from your recipes. You probably won't even notice it's gone! If you do, you can always add it on top of your food.

The reason it ended up being the easiest thing to give up, surprising no one more than myself, was that chicken really doesn't taste like anything, unless you add seasonings or sauce. I quickly found that whatever sauce I was putting over chicken, I could just as easily put over fish, a portabella mushroom, a baked potato, pasta or even steamed veggies. For example, a family favorite recipe for cranberry chicken quickly became cranberry portabellas, and it tastes *just* as good, because the flavor is all in the sauce, not in the chicken. After a few days of experimenting like this, I no longer missed chicken at all, and neither will you!

## assignment

Eliminate all poultry from your diet and your kitchen. (That food bank might be glad to see you again!) Try experimenting with your favorite chicken recipes by substituting fish, portabella mushrooms, baked potatoes or other food. Turn to your new collection of vegan recipes to find chicken alternatives.

# DAY
# 9

## add a large salad every day

If you have one really large salad every day, you will help your body get many important nutrients it needs to keep you healthy, and keep you full as well. Many people overeat all day long, yet are still nutrient deficient because they eat a diet almost entirely comprised of processed, packaged and fried foods, which are nearly devoid in vitamins and minerals. One way to help avoid this from happening to you is to make sure you're getting lots of nutrients in your diet. Adding a large salad to your diet every day is a great place to start.

Here is how to make a great vegan salad:

1. Start with a large bowl—even as large as a serving size bowl that you might use for a dinner party!

2. Fill the bowl with greens, preferably spinach, romaine or another dark leafy green. (Iceburg lettuce is practically devoid of nutrients.) An entire 5 ounce bag of greens is not too much.

3. Pile on fresh vegetables, fruits and beans, and sprinkle with a few nuts and seeds: corn, peas, avocado, cucumber, carrots, black beans, kidney beans, sprouts, bell peppers, tomatoes, raw almonds, raw sunflower seeds, jicama, beets, apples, mangoes, celery... you get the idea. If you use nuts and seeds, make sure they are 100% raw, and are not roasted or salted, for best health.

4. Top with a healthful salad dressing. Avoid all animal products, and try to steer clear of too much oil. There are some fantastic recipes for nut-based dressings and low-oil or no-oil vinaigrettes on the internet. You can also use hummus or a similar spread for your dressing instead of a traditional salad dressing. Look for low-calorie, low-fat dressings in your health food aisles, but read the ingredients carefully!

---

**tip**

A light drizzle of lemon juice or balsamic vinegar on your salad may be all you need for salad dressing. Don't forget to add freshly ground black pepper!

🍎

---

## assignment

From now on, eat one large salad every day. Start by getting yourself a large bowl that you love, if you don't already have one. Then, make a new salad every day for the next 7 days. Discover salads as if for the first time, and make them different each day. In the future, you'll have a lot of ideas for making salads from this one week of experimenting!

# DAY
# 10

## read *Diet for a New America*

Something made you pick up this book—something compelling. You may have bought this book to lose weight or become healthier, while another person may have bought it to help save the environment or reduce the suffering of animals. Whatever your reasons for picking up this book, you should understand all of the major arguments for veganism if you plan to eat this way, because people will expect you to know about them.

*Diet for a New America*, by John Robbins, is the one book that people have told me turned them on to veganism more than any other, and it was the book that convinced me to go vegan overnight. In fact, I was in an audience once when Mr. Robbins was about to speak, and the moderator asked the audience to raise their hand if John Robbins was the reason they had become vegetarian or vegan. About half the hands in the room went up, despite the fact that he was only one of about ten vegan speakers at the conference. His books are truly profound, and *Diet for a New America* is often considered his best work.

If you aren't interested in reading *Diet for a New America* to learn about all the aspects of veganism, then read it for this reason: It will likely motivate you to be vegan for life!

## assignment

Buy a copy of *Diet for a New America*, and read at least one chapter a day until you finish it. If financially feasible, buy a new or used copy rather than borrowing it from the library—you'll most certainly want to mark your copy up and keep it for further reference.

# DAY
# 11

## fruit and veg cleanse

Today you will do the second of your two fruit & veg cleanses. Notice that each cleanse occurs before you are eliminating a significant animal product from your diet—first meat, and now cheese. The cleanse should help you to adapt a little better to the elimination, especially psychologically, and should also help reduce your cravings for these foods.

---

### tip

Notice, specifically, how you feel after a day of eating only fruits and veggies. Do you have more energy? Need less sleep? Feel happier? You should feel fantastic during a cleanse!

---

Again, you should eat only organic raw fruits and veggies in their whole, natural form. Avoid anything canned, jarred or frozen.

After the 30-day program is over, you may want to do one fruit and veg cleanse day a week. Similarly, I often do a 3-day fruit and veg cleanse if I haven't been making wise food choices for a period of time—such as around the holidays—and I always feel amazing afterward.

## assignment

Eat only whole fruits and vegetables today, preferably raw, organic, and fresh from your grocer's produce section.

# DAY
# 12

## eliminate cheese

Starting today, you will eliminate all cheese from your diet and your kitchen. Cheese is just one of many dairy products, but it seems to be one of the bigger challenges for people to give up. According to Neal Barnard, MD, in his book, *Breaking the Food Seduction*, this is because cheese may be addictive. Dairy products contain casein, which break apart in digestion to release naturally occurring opiates called casomorphins. Astonishingly, casomorphins mimic the reaction of morphine on our brain! These opiates in dairy products may be responsible for the calming effect of nursing in infants, and perhaps for the addictive qualities in cheese!

Before I was vegan, and knew much about health, my four personal food groups were Swiss, Havarti, Cheddar and Chocolate. I ate more servings of dairy products—and especially cheese—than anything else. Macaroni and cheese was my favorite, followed by pasta with gorgonzola cheese sauce, and salad with ladles of blue cheese dressing. I was one of those people who really missed cheese when I first gave it up.

However, do you remember the "Big Secret" of veganism that I discussed on Day 4? Once you've cleansed your palate by avoiding all animal products, natural foods will begin to taste sublime, and your cravings for unhealthy foods will diminish and eventually go away. The cleaner you keep your diet—by not only avoiding animal products, but by also avoiding refined sugars, salt and added fats— the more your palate will be cleansed, and the less you will desire your old favorites. If you eat this way, you will truly enjoy eating healthfully, and will actually prefer *not* to eat unhealthy foods. Surprising no one more than myself, I now have absolutely no desire for cheese or chocolate; if I'm at a party and these items are near me, I hardly even notice they are there.

**tip**

My mom loves her cheese, and it's the one thing keeping her from a fully vegan diet. If you feel the same way about cheese, it will be essential to use non-vegan foods with a lot of flavor. For example, don't just make pasta with red sauce—add tangy sun-dried tomatoes, kalamata olives, marinated artichoke hearts and capers. This should give you enough flavor to make up for the lost cheese.

# assignment

Eliminate cheese from your diet and your kitchen. Notice that many foods, like burritos and pasta, are very good without all the cheese!

# DAY
# 13

# take a tour of your local health food store

Changing from the standard American diet to a natural foods diet can be a little daunting at first. When you go into a natural foods store, you won't find anything on the shelves from Nabisco, Kraft or General Mills. Instead, new brand names meet you, and products you've never heard of abound.

Don't despair! You'll notice right away that even though you can't find Cheerios, you can find Purely O's or some other natural version, which will usually taste the same, but without the chemical ingredients in it. The same thing holds true for salad dressings, frozen foods, and other items on your list. You'll simply have to try some new brands, and find out what you like.

Don't pressure yourself to understand the entire natural foods world right away. It was years before I tried cooking with nutritional yeast, knew what agave nectar was used for, or sprinkled stevia on my cereal. In fact, there are still many common natural food ingredients that I have never used.

Over time, you will read about these items in the natural foods store, and undoubtedly come across recipes that use them. In the meantime, if you want to buy convenience foods, feel free to stick with the items that look easiest to you—the natural versions of cereal, frozen burritos and soups. The fact that they aren't your usual brands is already a shock enough. Take it slowly, and never be afraid to ask questions of the store's staff.

Health food stores often have scheduled group tours, designed to help people new to the natural foods market understand the variety of different products. Smaller stores will sometimes offer individual tours instead, which is a nice personalized touch. If you'd like, you can take tours of all the different stores in your area that you think you might like to frequent!

## assignment

Call your local health food store and sign up for a store tour. After your tour, buy one new product that you have never tried before.

> **tip**
>
> Many traditional grocery stores now have separate natural foods sections, which is very handy. For today, however, go to a proper natural foods store for your tour, which will have a far wider range of products for you to learn about.

# DAY
# 14

## gather vegan recipes

One of the keys to making the vegan diet work is to make sure you have plenty of yummy, accessible vegan food around. If you only have a few dishes you like, you'll quickly get bored, and it will be hard to keep eating this way.

Fortunately, there are tons of incredible vegan recipes available... recipes so good, your carnivorous friends will be asking you for them! The key is to first track down vegan recipes, and then experiment with them to learn which ones you like best.

I recommend keeping a list or spreadsheet of all the recipes you make, where you found them (website address, specific cookbook and page, etc) and give them each a rating. Later, when you're having one of those days when you can't decide what to make for dinner, you can consult this spreadsheet, and even sort it by rating, so you can find just the dish that sounds great at that moment.

Here are some of my favorites:

## TRANSITION COOKBOOKS

These books are best when you are transitioning to a vegan diet, either because they have many of your old favorites made with vegan ingredients, and/or because they have a lot of flavor to them, making you wonder why you didn't go vegan years ago! Many of the recipes in these transition cookbooks will be healthy, but some will include oil, vegannaise (vegan mayonnaise) or other fatty, salty or sugary ingredients that I'd like you to eventually limit in your diet. Use your head, and choose accordingly!

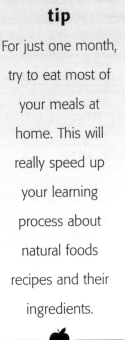

**tip**

For just one month, try to eat most of your meals at home. This will really speed up your learning process about natural foods recipes and their ingredients.

- *How it All Vegan!*
  – By Sarah Kramer and Tanya Barnard

- *The Garden of Vegan*
  – By Sarah Kramer and Tanya Barnard

- *Planet Vegan*
  – By Robin Robertson

## IDEAL COOKBOOKS

These cookbooks are ideal because they rely on whole foods, generally without added fats, salts and sugars. These foods will taste delicious to you in most cases, but if you're coming off a particularly fatty and greasy diet, you might miss the salt, sugar or fat. I use these resources almost exclusively now, and my husband and I generally love everything I make from them. The first two are cookbooks, and the second two are non-fiction books about health, with great recipe sections in the back.

- *Lorna Sass's Vegetarian Cooking Under Pressure*
  - By Lorna Sass
    *(In the rare event she adds cheese or another dairy product, just leave it out. Also, you will need a pressure cooker for these recipes, or will need to be confident enough to adapt it to a stove pot or slow cooker.)*

- *Kitchen in the Clouds*
  - By Karen Alexander and Suzanne Wood

- *Eat to Live*
  - By Joel Fuhrman, MD

- *Prevent & Reverse Heart Disease*
  - By Caldwell Esselstyn, MD

## WEBSITES

www.FatFreeVegan.com *(My #1 source for recipes!)*

www.DrFuhrman.com

www.DrMcDougall.com

www.VegSource.com

# assignment

Go to your local library or bookstore and look through the vegan cookbook section. Borrow or buy a book that looks good to you. Also go online and research vegan recipes.

# DAY
# 15

## try a new recipe

There is no doubt that learning to cook without meat, dairy and eggs means that you'll need to come up with a lot of new recipes. Yesterday you spent time gathering online recipes and researching vegan cookbooks. However, it's not just enough to gather the recipes—you have to actually make the food!

In my early months as a vegan, I found that if I didn't have enough variety of vegan food available to me, I became bored, and had a harder time adhering to the diet. To solve this problem, I committed to making at least one new dish a week for 52 weeks. This set me up with a great arsenal of recipes, and I always feel like I can make something quickly from my list that I know I'll like.

## assignment
Make one new vegan recipe today. Make a commitment to try at least one new recipe a week for the next 52 weeks.

# DAY
# 16

## eliminate fish and seafood

Starting today, you will eliminate all fish and seafood from your diet. You will also remove any fish and seafood products from your refrigerator, freezer and cupboards, and donate them or give them to a neighbor or family member. Don't forget about those cans of tuna lurking in the back of your cupboard!

In general, the hardest thing about giving up your last type of flesh product is that you feel you won't have any options left for your main entrée. It seems that all entrees revolve around meat, poultry or fish. However, there are so many options that don't include any of these products, as you've now learned from researching vegan recipes, that this should be one of those concerns you will learn to let go. This can seem a bit daunting when you eat out at restaurants, but you'll learn how to get around this on Day 25.

Just like poultry, what we generally like about eating fish is not the fish itself, but rather the sauce we put over it. You will quickly learn that you can re-create many of your favorite dishes by putting the same (or similar) sauces over vegetables or pasta instead. If you enjoy grilling your fish, and therefore, it's not necessarily the sauce you enjoy but rather the flavor from the grill, try grilling Portabella mushrooms instead. Not only can you re-create some of the same grill flavors using mushrooms, but they are also a great way to ease out of meat and fish products, because they have a fleshy consistency to them.

If you're used to using creamy or cheesy sauces, you should begin looking for sauces that don't include any animal products. Don't just settle for plain marinara sauce—add sundried tomatoes, kalamata olives, artichoke hearts and capers to it. Get creative! You can also make some fabulous pesto sauces (without parmesan,) and if you want to leave out the fat from the oil, you can create white bean pesto! Just look for the recipes in vegan cookbooks and on vegan websites.

## assignment

Eliminate all fish and seafood products from your diet and kitchen. Try experimenting with your favorite recipes by substituting portabella mushrooms, baked potatoes or pasta for the fish.

# DAY
# 17

## commit to the kitchen

In our fast-paced society, we love to be efficient—especially when it comes to cooking. This is undoubtedly why fast food, frozen foods and pre-packed dinners are so popular. It's very appealing to throw a frozen dinner into the microwave while you change into your sweats, and have dinner be hot and ready by the time you've changed!

However, this is simply not what's in the best interest of our health. Most processed food—food in boxes, bags, cans and jars—almost always contains added salt, sugar and fat, as well as harmful chemical additives. Many scientists believe that these tiny amounts of chemicals add up over the years, resulting in cancer for many of us.

If you are someone who likes to have dinner done in 5 minutes or less, yet still want to switch to a healthy vegan diet, it is to your advantage to commit a little more time to your kitchen. You don't need to spend hours slaving over the stove or growing your own organic garden, but cooking healthy food means cooking fresh food, so you will need to cook from time to time.

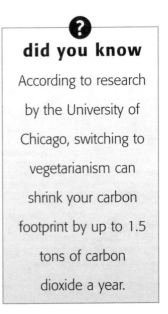

**did you know**

According to research by the University of Chicago, switching to vegetarianism can shrink your carbon footprint by up to 1.5 tons of carbon dioxide a year.

The good news, for those of you who don't like to spend much time in the kitchen, is that there are several strategies for shortening the time you spend in the kitchen.

For example, some of nature's best foods are grab and go items, which means you don't have to rely on convenience store items if you're in a hurry—it's just as easy to grab an apple or a banana (or both!) as you walk out the door in the morning, as it is to grab a Power Bar or doughnut at the gas station. If you're willing to add just a few extra minutes to your morning routine, you can reap tasty benefits. For example, with just a few more minutes, you can make some oatmeal with berries, or a fresh smoothie in your blender. Neither of these latter options is a grab and go item, but they don't take much time to prepare at all.

Another way to save time is by making one-pot meals. Many vegan recipes simply involve throwing all the ingredients into a soup pot, a crock pot, or a pressure cooker, and letting them cook. I always keep my eye out for these one-step recipes.

Finally, you can also save a lot of time in the kitchen by doubling and tripling recipes. If I'm making a batch of my favorite soup or my husband's favorite chili, I will double or triple the recipe—that leaves us with leftovers all week that I simply need to heat and serve. Then, dinner becomes just as fast as if I were heating up a microwave dinner!

If you want great health—and a slim waistline—it's in your best interest to commit to your kitchen. It doesn't have to be for hours a day, but committing to just a little more time each day is a simple decision that will change your health forever!

## assignment

Spend 20 minutes in your kitchen today, cutting fruit and vegetables for convenient snacking, or perhaps making a soup from scratch. Notice how great everything tastes when it's fresh and homemade!

# DAY
# 18

## buy a veggie chopper

As a vegan, there's really not many ways to get around the fact that you're going to have to chop veggies... a lot of veggies! As you just learned yesterday, you're going to need to spend some time in the kitchen.

To make this time shorter, one of the best investments you can make is in a veggie chopper. They are sold everywhere from Williams-Sonoma (Vegetable Chop and Measure) for about $30, to "As Seen on TV" (The Vidalia Chop Wizard) for about $20. Not only do they allow you to chop your veggies quickly, but unlike food processors, they are also a cinch to clean!

Here's how they work: With a veggie chopper, you put smallish pieces of veggies (for example, a quarter of an onion) onto a metal grate, and press the plastic lid down over the veggies, dicing them through the grate. The diced veggies go into a plastic, graduated container, instantly allowing you to measure how much you've just diced. Brilliant!

## assignment

Get online or go to your local cooking store, and buy a veggie chopper. As soon as you get one, cut an onion into 4 equal pieces, and then dice the pieces with your new chopper. See just how fast (and generally tear free) this chore has become!

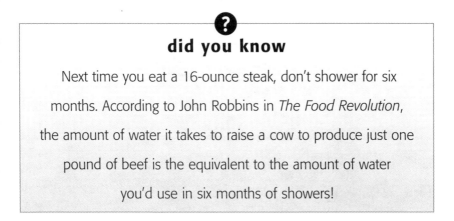

### ❓ did you know

Next time you eat a 16-ounce steak, don't shower for six months. According to John Robbins in *The Food Revolution*, the amount of water it takes to raise a cow to produce just one pound of beef is the equivalent to the amount of water you'd use in six months of showers!

# DAY
# 19

## treat yourself!

It's fun to be a vegan, and thanks to superstars like Alicia Silverstone, Shania Twain and Carl Lewis, it's now hip to be vegan, too!

You can show your vegan pride by purchasing one of the many t-shirts, mugs, or even pairs of underwear that advertise your new vegan status. If you prefer to be more low-key, how about buying a pair of shoes or an outfit—with no animal products used in their production? Perhaps you'd like to splurge on a book about the vegan diet? Whatever strikes your fancy, today is a day to treat yourself.

## assignment

Treat yourself to something that is vegan-related. Spend as little or as much as you'd like! You can find an amazing selection of vegan pride items at **www.cafepress.com**. You can also google vegan clothing and shoes, and you can search for vegan books online too. Have fun!

# DAY
# 20

## eliminate eggs

Starting today, you will eliminate eggs from your diet and your kitchen. The two most common places to find eggs in your meals are either as a main item, like scrambled eggs, or as an ingredient in baked goods.

If you like eggs for breakfast, you can make scrambled tofu, which is surprisingly delicious, and you'll still get plenty of protein. Unfortunately, I have not come across a substitute for hard-boiled or fried eggs. In this case, perhaps you can try switching to scrambled tofu, or finding a completely different food, like oatmeal, to take it's place.

Baked goods are the other common place to find eggs, and if you enjoy baking, you'll have to find substitutes for eggs. There are

> **tip**
>
> Many types of pasta are simply made from durum semolina. Penne pasta is one of these, and is almost always a sure bet for egg-free pasta.

a number of substitutes for eggs in baking, and sometimes, you can try simply leaving the eggs out of a recipe altogether! My husband was recently yearning for cornbread; in a hurry and not particularly adept at baking, I decided to eliminate the egg in the recipe without replacing it with another binder, and the result was absolutely fine! Here are some tips that I found at **www.pcrm.org** for egg substitutes:

- If a recipe calls for just one or two eggs, you can often skip them. Add a couple of extra tablespoons of water for each egg eliminated to balance out the moisture content of the product.

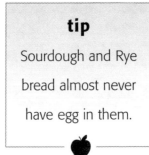

**tip**

Sourdough and Rye bread almost never have egg in them.

- Eggless egg replacers are available in many natural food stores. These are different from reduced-cholesterol egg products, which do contain eggs. Egg replacers are egg-free and are usually in a powdered form. Replace eggs in baking with a mixture of the powdered egg replacer and water according to package directions.

- Use 1 heaping tablespoon of soy flour or cornstarch plus 2 tablespoons of water to replace each egg in a baked product.

- Use 1 ounce of mashed tofu in place of an egg.

- In muffins and cookies, half of a mashed banana can be used instead of an egg, although it will change the flavor of the recipe somewhat.

- For vegetarian loaves and burgers, use any of the following to bind ingredients together: tomato paste, mashed potato, moistened breadcrumbs, or rolled oats.

If you are like me, and don't like to bake, but do love eating baked goods, you'll need to find places that sell vegan baked goods. Natural food stores and supermarkets that have a health food aisle are usually good places to find these items. The better health food stores and bakeries make delicious vegan cakes, cookies, scones and even donuts! I'm sure they are not particularly healthful, but if you need a sweet fix, you'll know exactly where to go!

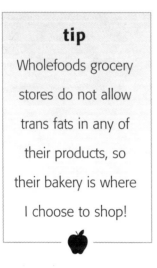

**tip**

Wholefoods grocery stores do not allow trans fats in any of their products, so their bakery is where I choose to shop!

The tricky thing about eliminating eggs is that they are ubiquitous: Not only are they a common ingredient in products that you buy on the shelves of your grocery store, but they are also included in some restaurant foods, particularly in bread products.

You'll have to get used to reading labels when you're at the grocery store, and make a point of not buying products that include eggs. When you're at restaurants, you can decide how much you plan to "investigate." The most obvious solution is to tell your waiter that you're vegan, and ask him about each item you're considering, to ensure there are no animal products in them. That is my general approach. Some vegans, however, simply order items that would normally not have animal products in them, so they can avoid making a fuss. For example, unless you are eating at an authentic Italian restaurant where they make all of their pasta from scratch, it's a pretty safe bet that fettuccine pasta will have egg in it, but penne pasta won't. You could order penne pasta with a red puttanesca sauce, and be fairly sure it's vegan. My personal opinion is that I go out to eat to be waited on, so I'm not shy about asking for exactly what I want. There is more about eating out at restaurants in Chapter 25.

## assignment

Eliminate eggs from your diet and your kitchen. If you enjoy baking, try making some recipes that use a substitute for eggs. If you like to buy baked goods, find some local places that carry vegan baked goods, and try one of their products. Finally, the next time you go out to dinner, order something that won't include eggs—and avoid the bread basket unless you get a specific thumbs up from your waiter!

**tip**

Eating eggs for their protein? Don't worry about it anymore! Broccoli has more protein per pound than sirloin steak. It's a myth that vegans can't get enough protein.

# DAY
# 21

## meet other vegans

Sometimes it can be a little daunting to be vegan. Some cities have huge communities of them, but residents in some small towns aren't even sure what a vegan is! Wherever you live, you can meet other vegans—either in person or online. Knowing other vegans—even if only virtual acquaintances—makes it easier to stay on track, especially at this key time of transition. It's nice to have friends that understand what you're doing, and who you can call on for help, suggestions, motivation, and recipes.

If you'd like to meet people in person, my first suggestion is to go online and look for vegan groups in your area. One website, **www.MeetUp.com**, organizes meetings for people in your area with all kinds of specific interests—even vegan! Another way to meet vegans is to go to meetings of environmental and animal rights organizations—most people in these groups tend to be vegan or vegetarian. You can also go to your local vegan restaurants and natural food stores and look on their post-it boards for any groups that are advertising meetings.

If you'd prefer to just meet a few people online, your options are endless. **www.VeggieBoards.com** is filled with vegans and vegetarians that chat back and forth. **www.VegSource.com** is another option for meeting fellow vegans. Some doctors that promote a vegan or near vegan diet have a lot of vegans on their forums discussing health and recipe issues. Try **www.DrFurhman.com** or **www.DrMcDougall.com**, among others. Animal rights and environmental groups also have forums where people chat, and of course, there are vegan and vegetarian singles' forums on the web too. Just jump online and start searching!

## assignment

Meet at least one new vegan today, either online or in person. If you need more time to meet people in person, then use today to make a specific plan for when you're going to meet up with a vegan group.

**DAY**

# 22

## stay motivated!

The absolute best way that I've found to stay motivated to eat a vegan diet in the long-term is to simply continue to learn about it. After you have read, watched and heard a critical amount of information (that amount is different for everyone,) you will probably be motivated for life. You may have already reached this point, or you may be close—you never know until you've reached it! Usually, one thing you read or hear will be the item that tips you over the edge into committing to a vegan diet forever.

If you are not currently committed to being vegan forever, but would really like to be, simply keep engrossing yourself in vegan material; eventually you won't be able to help but decide to go vegan forever. The arguments—from almost every angle—are simply too strong.

If you have committed to being a life-long vegan, you may still find yourself in need of motivation from time to time—especially to keep eating a healthy vegan diet, and not succumbing to a diet of fries and soda. I find that I need additional motivation to eat a healthy vegan diet about twice a year. When I see my healthy habits starting to slip, I pick up the latest book or order the newest vegan DVD. Retreats and online support groups can really be a fun way to stay motivated, and are extremely effective. This is your health: invest in it! A vegan retreat may seem pricey, but it will probably cost a lot less than your medical bills if you go back to eating the standard American diet.

Finally, to motivate yourself not only to eat a vegan diet, but also to succeed in all areas of your life, don't let another day go by without listening to the CDs of some of the best motivational speakers in the world. My absolute favorite is Tony Robbins, although there are so many great speakers to choose from. Go to your library and borrow CDs by Tony Robbins, Zig Ziglar, Brian Tracy, Jim Rohn and others. Your life will never be the same again!

---

### tip
www.Vegsource.com hosts a weekend seminar
every year in the LA area with all the top speakers
in the area of veganism and health. Plan to attend, or order
a past year's DVD set and watch it at home.
The information at these retreats is astounding!

---

The following pages list the best vegan resources I have found to keep me motivated. I'm sure this is only the tip of the iceberg, so have fun cruising the bookstores and the web, finding even more. Enjoy!

# BOOKS

*Diet for a New America*, by John Robbins

*The Food Revolution*, by John Robbins

*Healthy at 100*, by John Robbins

*The China Study*, by T. Colin Campbell, PhD

*Eat to Live*, by Joel Fuhrman, MD

*Green for Life*, by Victoria Boutenko

*Vegan: The Ethics of Eating*, by Erik Marcus

*Breaking the Food Seduction*, by Neal Barnard, MD

*Prevent and Reverse Heart Disease*,
by Caldwell Esselstyn, MD

*The Pleasure Trap*,
by Doug Lisle, PhD and Alan Goldhammer, PhD

*Slaughterhouse*, by Gail Eisnitz

*Plant Roots*, by Rex Bowlby

*The 12-Day McDougall Diet*, by John McDougall, MD

*Diet for a Small Planet*, by Francis Moore-Lappe

*Thrive*, by Brendan Brazier

*The Great American Detox Diet*, by Alex Jamieson

*The Vegan Handbook*, by Deborah Wasserman

## WEBSITES

www.BeautifulOnRaw.com

www.cafepress.com

www.DrFuhrman.com

www.DrMcDougall.com

www.HarmonyEarth.net

www.PETA.org

www.PCRM.org

www.rawfoods.com

www.TrueFoodNow.org

www.vegan.com

www.VeggieBoards.com

www.VegSource.com

www.VRG.org

**tip**

The works of the best motivational speakers in the world are nearly all conglomerated in one place: **www.nightingaleconant.com**. This site is a fantastic resource for all things motivational.

## assignment

Hopefully, you're finding that this book is motivating you right now toward your goal of becoming a vegan. However, be prepared for the end of this program by researching a new motivational speaker, online vegan doctor or other source from the list above, so that you will have another place to turn to for motivation when this 30-day program is over.

# DAY
# 23

## begin taking vitamin B12 and ground flaxseed

Vitamin B12 is the only nutrient that is not readily found in the westernized vegan diet. We need trace amounts of Vitamin B12 in the diet for proper nerve and brain function, and vitamin B12 is found in meat products.

Does this imply that the vegan diet is lacking, and perhaps we *should* be eating non-vegan foods? The answer is "no." Here's why: Vitamin B12 does not *originate* in animal products; Vitamin B12 originates in the soil. When we eat vegetables in today's modern society (as opposed to when we were cavemen) we wash our veggies thoroughly—almost obsessively. Without bits of soil left on our veggies, we don't ingest any of that soil, and we therefore don't ingest any Vitamin B12. Cows and many other animals, however, eat grass, ripping it out at the roots, and they do ingest the soil, thus ingesting Vitamin B12 along with it. This B12 gets assimilated into their muscles, fat and organs. Then, when we eat beef, for example, we ingest the B12 from their flesh. That is how most people get their B12 in today's society.

As a vegetarian or vegan, you should take a Vitamin B12 supplement. I recommend taking a sublingual (under the tongue) tablet, which absorbs into your body more efficiently than swallowing a pill. The Recommended Daily Intake (RDI) for vitamin B12 is only 6 mcg, so buy the smallest dose available. You should be able to find sublingual vitamin B12 at most drugstores and supermarkets. I get mine from Trader Joes.

Your body only needs trace amounts of B12, and it takes a long time to build and a long time to lose your reserves. It's estimated that vegans who quit eating meat and don't take any supplements for B12 will lose the B12 stores in their bodies in about 3 to 5 years' time. If this happens, you might notice tingling in your fingers and/or toes, dizziness, or other nervous system symptoms. While this would be considered somewhat rare, it's not worth risking, so just take your B12 tablets!

In addition to vitamin B12, vegans also need to ensure they get enough omega-3 fatty acids in their diet. Studies have shown that omega-3's help boost your immune function, reverse heart disease, improve fertility, promote good mental health and help fight degenerative diseases.

> **tip**
>
> Many ethnic restaurants serve a lot of vegetarian and vegan food because they are from countries where the religion prohibits eating meat. Asian restaurants will especially offer a large variety of vegetarian and vegan options for this reason.

Our ancestors got plenty of omega 3's by eating wild plants and wild game. However, as John Robbins points out in his book *Healthy at 100*, in modern society, we don't eat wild plants, and modern meat and dairy products contain greatly reduced levels of this important nutrient.

The main source for omega-3's in the westernized diet is fish. Sadly, almost all the fish we consume comes from fish farms, and studies show that these fish are polluted with toxic chemicals and pollutants like methyl mercury, PCBs dioxins, and banned insecticides. These toxins can affect your central nervous system, your autoimmune system, and can cause cancers and birth defects. Obviously, these are not ingredients we want to ingest!

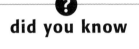

**did you know**

According to Joel Fuhrman, MD in *Eat to Live*, a person would have to drink the water in the Great Lakes for 100 years to accumulate the same quantity of PCBs in a half-pound portion of trout or salmon from these lakes.

Fortunately, there is a good vegan source for omega-3s, and that is flaxseeds. Because the shells of flaxseeds prevent the nutrients from being readily available for absorption, the best way to get the omega-3s out of the flaxseed is to either grind it or take it in oil form. I grind up a cup of flaxseed or so in a coffee grinder, and sprinkle a tablespoon on my breakfast every morning. You can also blend it into your smoothies, use it as a soup topping, or sprinkle it on salads and other foods.

Alternately, you can take 1-2 tablespoons of flaxseed oil every day. Like B12, omega-3s are very important for a healthy body, so don't ignore this advice—take your flaxseed every day!

# assignment

Go to your health food store and get some vitamin B12 sublingual tablets. Also get some fresh flaxseed (it will probably be in the refrigerated bulk section) or flaxseed oil. Start taking both today!

# DAY
# 24

## eliminate all dairy

Starting today, you will eliminate all dairy products from your diet and your kitchen. By this time, you've already given up cheese, so eliminating the rest of the dairy aisle hopefully won't be too much of a struggle—especially since there are so many substitutes available. The most obvious dairy products that are left to give up are milk, ice cream, creamy dressings, yogurt, sour cream and butter.

**tip**

The Native Foods Cookbook has an incredible recipe for vegan Ranch Dressing in it.

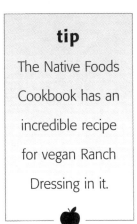

Like almost everything we are eliminating from our diet, there are a lot of vegan substitutes for these dairy products—many are listed back in Day 5, for your reference. You'll probably need to go to a health food store or find a supermarket with a good health food aisle to find some of them. Since you've already gone on a tour of your local health food store, you may have already found many of them.

There are great vegan substitutes and recipes for sour cream, creamy dressings (even Caesar dressing!) and ice cream. Make sure you try different brands, as we already discussed. I have found some incredible soy-based ice creams that I adore, but some other brands leave a funny aftertaste to me. Try soymilk in place of regular milk, and if you like butter, try one of the vegan "heart-healthy" butter substitutes. Many times you may be able to substitute oil or even water for butter, such as when sautéing vegetables. You can also use margarine, which is vegan, but it's not a healthy alternative due to the trans fats found in it, so use it only as a last resort.

## assignment

Eliminate all dairy items from your diet and your kitchen. Go to the store and buy a vegan version of a regular dairy product you might otherwise have bought. Alternately, try making the vegan version of a recipe that would normally have dairy in it.

# DAY
# 25

## learn to eat in restaurants

People love to eat out at restaurants. It's social, it's convenient, and it's just plain yummy... even as a vegan! If you live in a larger city, you may have several vegan restaurants to choose from—divine! But if you live in a smaller city or town, you may not be so lucky. That's okay! Almost every restaurant has vegan items on the menu already, or if not, you can easily create them with a little ingenuity and a special request for the chef. I never have problems eating vegan in restaurants. Furthermore, my food usually looks so much better than everyone else's that they make comments about wishing they had what I was having! Here are some specific suggestions for eating out at non-vegan restaurants.

1. **Call ahead.** Ask them to tell the chef that you are vegan, and tell them when you'll be dining there. They will appreciate the heads-up, and you will probably get a better meal, since the chef will have had time to think about it. Don't forget to tell them specifically what vegans *don't* eat, just in case they think vegans are the same as vegetarians.

2. **Scan the menu for vegan items.** Pasta primavera, vegetarian sushi or stir-fry noodles with veggies and tofu are all popular options. Salads with a vinaigrette dressing are always a good stand-by, and have become very interesting and delicious over the years.

3. **Tell them what you want—even if it's nowhere on the menu.** If fruit is not on the menu for dessert, ask for it anyway—chances are you'll get it. If pasta primavera is nowhere to be found on the menu, ask for it anyway—chances are you'll get it. You get the idea!

4. **Look for easy substitutions.** For example, the Chinese Chicken Salad without the chicken, or a vegetarian burrito without the sour cream and cheese. You'd be surprised at what tastes great, even without cheese, meat or butter!

5. **Look for options from non-vegan items that you can combine to make vegan.** For example, if the menu has Spaghetti Bolognese, and Chicken with Vegetables, ask for Spaghetti with Vegetables. You can also look at all the different side dishes that come with the main entrees, and ask the waiter to make you a full meal of different vegan side dishes.

6. **Ask the chef to make you something on his or her own.** This is one of my favorite options because I often get the most delicious dinners if I just let the chef get creative. This is almost a guaranteed winner in better restaurants, but in cheap restaurants, beware: you could end up with white rice and steamed vegetables, with no flavor at all. Don't be afraid to tell them what you don't want!

## assignment

Go out to eat tonight, or make plans to eat out on the weekend. You can call ahead, if you'd like, or just show up at one of your favorite places and see what you can find or adapt on the menu.

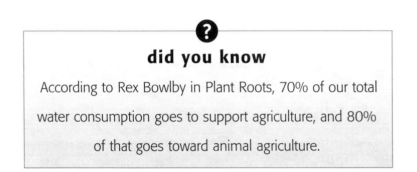

### ❓ did you know

According to Rex Bowlby in Plant Roots, 70% of our total water consumption goes to support agriculture, and 80% of that goes toward animal agriculture.

# DAY
# 26

## attending and hosting dinner parties

Many people will want to invite you over to dinner or a party, yet may be nervous about what to cook for you. I have a general rule of thumb: since it takes a lot of effort to host a dinner or party, I don't want to add to the hostess's stress by having her cook something separately for me. Therefore, I follow these guidelines when I am asked over for dinner:

1. First, if the hostess has not acknowledged that I am a vegan, and I think she either may not know, or may have forgotten, I make sure to tell her when I RSVP. However…

2. I *always* make sure I offer to bring my own dish. In fact, I specifically say that since she will have a lot of other cooking to do, I would be happy to bring my own dish, with enough for everyone for share. I tell the hostess that many of my other friends have me bring my own dish when I come to dinner, implying that this is how my other friends deal with my diet, and thus, it's perfectly acceptable for her to do the same. Then, if she agrees to let me bring my own dish, I make something really

delicious like veggie ceviche, that is a complete meal for me, and also yummy for everyone else as a side dish. If you bring a fabulous dish, chances are that people will be more open to learning about the vegan diet—you've just shown them that vegan food isn't horrible like they may have assumed!

3. If the hostess absolutely insists on doing the cooking, then I try to make it very easy. I tell her that I usually just eat salad with vinaigrette dressing, some bread on the side, and some veggies without sauce. Chances are she was planning to make some version of these foods anyway, so I'm not putting her out too much. Then I offer to bring the bread; that way I can make sure it doesn't contain butter or eggs.

4. If the hostess is really relishing the challenge of making a true vegan meal, then I just oblige and tell her what vegans eat and don't eat. Then I let her have fun, and enjoy the treat!

Sometimes, you will be the one hosting a dinner or party, and you'll need to think ahead about what you'd like to do. Will you allow all types of food in your house? If so, make a great meal or hors d'ouvres that have both non-vegan and vegan options. Make sure you include several vegan dishes, as people will be curious about your diet, and will want to try vegan food. Be sure to make your best recipes, though, to show them that vegan food can be really delicious! You can guarantee that most people will be skeptical; this is your chance to abolish their skepticism.

If you would rather that your house be 100% vegetarian or 100% vegan, make sure your guests know this ahead of time. Obviously this is crucial if you are having a potluck. Even if you're not, people may bring milk chocolates, smoked salmon or other gifts of food, and you wouldn't want to embarrass them if they found out that you keep a vegan or vegetarian house.

My husband and I only eat vegan in our house, but allow vegetarian food in the house if guests come over. If we have a potluck or dinner party, we let everyone know that we keep a vegetarian house for guests, and ask them only to bring vegetarian or vegan foods. Since vegetarian food includes eggs and dairy products, it is easy to accommodate, so most people are quite comfortable with that.

## assignment

Invite a non-vegan friend or couple to your house for dinner this week. Spend time today researching recipes and deciding what you will make. Either make a few vegan dishes for them to try, or make an entire vegan dinner... from start to finish!

# DAY
# 27

## learn how to say,
## "no thank you, i'm vegan"

As we near the end of our 30-day plan, I am going to arm you with two very important skills: the ability to say "no," and the ability to explain your stance on the vegan diet when people question you. Today, we are going to focus on simply saying "no."

As a vegan, there will be many times when you need to say, "no, thank you,"… as a waiter comes to grate cheese over your meal, as a salesperson offers you a free sample, or perhaps most uncomfortably, when a friend makes a special non-vegan dish for you.

Hopefully, you will find it easy to simply say, "No, thank you," if a waiter or stranger offers you a non-vegan item. There is no need to pronounce your vegan ideals in this case. A simple smile of appreciation, along with a sincere, "No, but thank you for offering," should be enough. If you have the type of personality that has a very difficult time saying "no," you will need to work on this. You can start by going to Costco and politely declining all the free samples! Another way to graciously say no is with a beaming smile: If the girl scouts come by and ask if you'd like to buy cookies, put a big smile on your face and say, "No thank you, but good luck! I know you'll sell a lot of those!" By smiling and wishing a person good luck, you leave them on an upbeat note, and they won't feel defeated.

A bit more disconcerting is the situation when someone makes you a non-vegan dish, either on accident, or because they don't realize that you're vegan.

There should really never be a case when someone makes you a non-vegan dish because they don't realize you're vegan. You should always remember to either bring your own food or call ahead and warn the chef or hostess about your food preferences. You would do this if you had a severe peanut allergy, wouldn't you?

If, on the very rare occasion when you unexpectedly end up someplace where the hostess wasn't expecting you and didn't know you were vegan, simply take her aside early and say, "I don't want to cause you any trouble, but I wanted to let you know that I eat a vegan diet, so I won't be having any chicken tonight. However, the green beans, salad and rice look absolutely delicious, so if it's okay with you, I'll just have those." Catching your hostess ahead of time will help to avoid a scene at the dinner table, and will make your hostess more comfortable. Better yet, if the meal will be served family or buffet style, you may never even have to mention your diet to her—if there are vegan options available, you can simply pile your plate with the vegan items and she'll probably never notice. Remember that good manners are simply a matter of making the people around you comfortable.

A much trickier situation is when someone makes you a non-vegan dish because they forgot you were vegan, or because they didn't really understand the extent of the vegan diet when they made the recipe.

One time, a good friend was having a dinner party for eight people, and went out of her way to make several vegan dishes for me. Her crowning glory was her apple pie—she had made one regular version and one vegan version... or so she thought! I was very touched that she had made me a vegan pie, and was, quite honestly, astounded by it. I said to her, "Oh my gosh—I can't believe you did this for me! I didn't even know you could make a pie without using milk, butter or eggs!" All of a sudden, her smile faded, and she was clearly crestfallen; in her efforts to substitute milk and eggs, she had forgotten that butter wasn't allowed, and her efforts were for naught.

In this very touchy situation, many people would argue that I should have eaten a little bit anyway. After all, my friend had gone to so much effort, peeling apples with her kids into the wee hours of the night, and no one else wanted a near-vegan pie! I understand this point of reasoning, and if veganism was purely a personal preference for me, I probably would have done just that. However, because I am a vegan for ethical reasons, I have a personal policy that I will never knowingly eat animal products. I believe that one of my roles is to set an example for others and to live out my values in public. Therefore, there was never a question in my mind as to whether I would eat the pie. The question was how to best handle the situation.

When my friend's face fell upon realizing her mistake—and undoubtedly realizing that all those hours were wasted—I put my arms around her and gave her a big, big hug. I then looked her in the eye and told her that the fact that she would go to so much effort for me meant even more than the pie itself, and that her gesture was one of the kindest that anyone had ever shown me. I also pointed out that she had made so many vegan dishes for me to eat, that I would probably never have room for pie anyway! This made her smile, and helped to cheer her up.

The next time we were invited to her house for dinner, she once again made me several vegan dishes. At the end of the night, she pulled two apple pies out of the oven—one regular pie, and one that was truly vegan! And it was the best apple pie I ever ate.

## assignment

When you are alone in your house or car, imagine showing up at a friend's house who accidentally made you a non-vegan dish. Practice what you would say to her, *out loud*, until you have your answer perfected. Make sure you practice not only what you would say, but also the actual facial expressions and gestures you would use as well. This may sound a little silly, but you'll be so glad you practiced when you come across this situation for the first time!

# DAY
# 28

## eliminate remaining animal ingredients

Starting today, you will eliminate all remaining animal ingredients from your diet and your kitchen. You may be asking what is left that you haven't already taken out! Well, there are a lot of minor ingredients that show up on food labels that are made from animal products, but we may not recognize them as animal products. For example, if you see an ingredient with the prefix "lact-" such as lactic acid or lactose, it almost undoubtedly comes from milk. Other ingredients are trickier, because they don't have a common prefix to look for, but they still come from animal sources—a few great examples are acetate, casein and whey. Finally, others are downright sneaky: "Natural flavors" often come from animal sources, and because the USDA does not require manufacturers to disclose the specific natural flavors, there is no way of knowing if animal products are present unless you call the manufacturer!

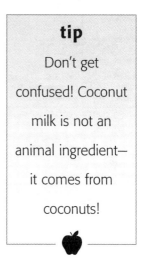

**tip**

Don't get confused! Coconut milk is not an animal ingredient— it comes from coconuts!

74

Here is a partial list of some of the more common animal ingredients that you may not have known came from animals:

## COMMON NON-VEGAN INGREDIENTS
▼

Acetate

Albumin

Casein

Fatty Acids

Gelatin

Glycerin

Lactose, most ingredients with the prefix "lact-"

Lanolin

Lard

Lecithin
(unless specified as soy lecithin)

Lipase, most ingredients with the prefix "lip-"

Milk Protein

Milk Sugar

Natural Flavoring
(often comes from animal sources)

Natural Sources
(often comes from animal sources)

Olean/Olestra

Palmitate

Rennin

Retinol

RNA/DNA

Stearic Acid

Stearyl Alcohol

Sterol

Whey

## assignment

Today you will eliminate all remaining non-vegan ingredients from your diet and your kitchen. Learn about non-vegan ingredients by either researching them online, or by buying a book that lists them. I highly recommend a short booklet called, *Animal Ingredients A to Z*, by E. G. Smith Collective.

# DAY
# 29

## clean out your kitchen

Now that you have educated yourself on the vegan diet, you are going to go through your kitchen and ensure that everything left is 100% vegan. You should have already donated or thrown out all non-vegan items through the course of the last 28 days, but there may be some last items that you have forgotten about, or that were hidden in the back of your pantry or freezer.

If you live with non-vegans who are not yet ready to eat this way with you, designate a separate shelf in the

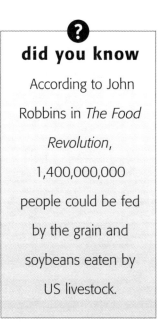

**did you know**

According to John Robbins in *The Food Revolution*, 1,400,000,000 people could be fed by the grain and soybeans eaten by US livestock.

refrigerator and a separate shelf in the pantry for your foods. Then you will know exactly which areas are yours. Keep an eye on your food though! Over time, you may find some of it missing, when they start snacking on your wonderful vegan food!

## assignment

Go through your kitchen and throw out all of the non-vegan items. If your cupboards are a bit empty, go to the store, and stock up on fruits, veggies, beans, grains, nuts and seeds.

# DAY
# 30

## state your case

As a vegan, people will naturally be intrigued about why you have chosen to eat this way. Those of us who have done it for a while find it very easy, but for those eating the standard American diet, it might seem excessively strict. People will ask you questions—some because they are curious, some because they are concerned about your health, and others because they are being aggressive and argumentative—and you must be able to state your case eloquently and confidently for choosing the vegan diet. Most importantly, you must be able to state your case without getting defensive!

People you know will undoubtedly want to know why you are choosing to eat a vegan diet. Unless they seem hostile about it (in which case, read further on,) just assume they are truly intrigued, and just want to know why. Don't get defensive or worry that they are being critical— they probably aren't. Most are just truly fascinated. Simply tell them what you've learned that has convinced you to make this big change in your life.

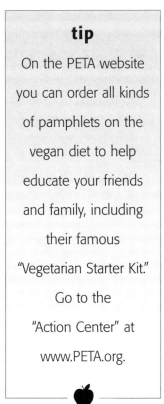

**tip**

On the PETA website you can order all kinds of pamphlets on the vegan diet to help educate your friends and family, including their famous "Vegetarian Starter Kit." Go to the "Action Center" at www.PETA.org.

Some friends and family may be concerned for your health; it's common for people to think that the vegan diet is deficient in protein or calcium, for example. In this case, you can try to explain all the information that will appease their worry, or you can give them a short answer, and then direct them to books for more information. You may even want to get brochures that you can hand out to people to educate them and assuage their fears.

The last group of people who may question you about your diet are the aggressive, argumentative types. Many people have very strong opinions about diet, animal rights activists, and environmentalists, and will likely attack you about your views—or what they assume are your views. Unfortunately, some people not only like to start arguments, but also like to start them in front of others, putting you in a very uncomfortable situation indeed! I find that the best way to handle this type of person is to give them a sincere smile to disarm them, and then give your 1-2 sentence reply about why you chose to eat a vegan diet (which you'll learn about on the next page.) Then, quickly change the subject by asking them something about themselves that is on a different subject. If they persist, answer their questions as succinctly and as kindly as you can; if they continue to push you, simply say, "Well, I appreciate what you're saying, but based on what I've read, I believe this is the right decision for me." Repeat this sentence as many times as you need, without adding more, until they quit attacking you. Most importantly, do not fall for their trap and get defensive. You have no reason to defend anything!

As you know, there is a lot of information about the vegan diet and several reasons why people choose it. When people ask you why you chose to adopt a vegan diet, it's tempting to try to relay all the information you have learned at once. However, this is very hard to do, and you will probably do more harm than good if you try cover everything at once. I suggest having your 1-2 sentence reply, and your 60-second "elevator speech."

Use your one to two sentence reply when the person asking just seems to be making small talk, and doesn't really appear to want a long answer. I use this one:

"Well, I originally started eating this way for animal welfare and environmental reasons, but then I also learned how incredibly healthy the vegan diet is, and that is now another major reason I eat this way."

Another option might be, "Well, I've read an incredible amount of scientific information about diet and nutrition, and have become convinced that this is the healthiest diet for humans." Period. No need to elaborate.

In other situations, people are looking to start a conversation about your diet. Many people will be very curious about why you eat a vegan diet—especially if you don't fit their preconceived notion of what a vegan looks like! Many people associate vegans with Berkeley students wearing tie-dyes, so if you don't fit that mold, they are truly interested in why *you* are vegan! For these people, I recommend having a 15-45 second "elevator speech"—a short reply that you could give in the time it takes for an elevator ride—to get the conversation rolling. Since you have a little more time, I recommend touching on a few subjects to peak their interest—hopefully baiting them to ask more! Here's what I say:

"Well, I originally started eating this way for animal welfare and environmental reasons, but then I also learned how incredibly healthy the vegan diet is, and that is now another major reason I eat this way. For example, did you know that Americans consume among the highest amounts of dairy products in the world, yet we also have among the highest rates of osteoporosis? Believe it or not, many scientists are now linking dairy products with osteoporosis, and the vegan diet doesn't include any dairy products. Similarly, many studies have linked animal proteins to cancer, but plant proteins don't seem to have the same cancer-causing effects. There are so many reasons why I eat a vegan diet, I could go on for hours…"

Usually their interest is peaked enough that they ask me to go on, or they say, "What do you mean, dairy products can cause osteoporosis!?" Thus, they are inviting me to continue the conversation.

If you are like me, and can read information about a subject and know it in your head, but not always be able to relay it eloquently when someone asks, you'll need to practice your answers out loud. It's much better to practice in your car than to practice on skeptics, who may be looking for ways to poke holes in your reasoning. If you haven't practiced what you're going to say, they'll probably find many holes!

> **tip**
>
> If you sometimes have a hard time expressing yourself eloquently to other people, try joining Toastmasters. Toastmasters is a non-profit club that helps people learn to speak in public. It's not only great for answering questions about your diet—it will be great for your career, too!

# assignment

When you are alone in your house or car, practice both your 1-2 sentence answer, as well as your 60-second elevator speech, about why you eat a vegan diet. Practice *out loud* until you have your answers nailed. Remember, smiling always softens people, so if you expect someone may get hostile, practice smiling when you give your responses!

"It's not that some people have willpower and some don't. It's that some people are ready to change, and others are not."

— *James Gordon, MD*

———— 🍎 ————

# celebration!

Congratulations! If you have taken the steps outlined throughout this book, you should now be a healthy vegan—or at least a vegan who is on his or her way to becoming healthy! Maybe you did this program in 30 days, or maybe it took you longer. The important thing is that you kept persisting with your goal and you made it through. My favorite definition of success is this:

### SUCCESS
**The progressive realization of a worthy ideal.**

The fact that you have taken steps over the past 30 or more days to progressively realize the worthy ideal of veganism, makes you a success. For that, I congratulate you, and hope that you are very proud of your accomplishment!

"One of the very nicest things about life
is the way we must regularly stop whatever it is
we are doing and devote our attention to eating."

— *Luciano Pavarotti*

# recipes

The following pages contain some of my favorite recipes to get you started on a vegan diet. I don't like to spend a lot of time in the kitchen, but I love to eat good food, so you'll find these recipes easy to make, yet full of flavor. You'll notice that I've left plenty of room at the bottom of each page for you to make notes on what you like, or how you might change the recipe in the future.

By now you've come across dozens of recipes in cookbooks and on the internet. Keep trying new recipes over the next year or so, and don't forget to print them out and keep track of the ones you like best. Over time, you'll be thrilled with all of the new dishes in your cooking repertoire! Enjoy!

# tropical green smoothie

## ingredients

- 1 Bag of Frozen Tropical Fruit Blend *(make sure the ingredients list only 100% whole fruit)*

- 2 C Water

- 1 - 2 Large Handfuls of Spinach

## prepare

Put water and spinach in a Vitamix or other high-powered blender, followed by the frozen fruit. Blend until smooth. Makes about 32 oz.

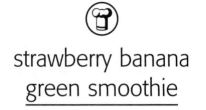

# strawberry banana
# green smoothie

## ingredients

- ◯ 1 Banana
- ◯ 1 C Frozen Strawberries
- ◯ 2 C Water
- ◯ 1 Bunch Romaine

## prepare

Put water and romaine lettuce in a Vitamix or other high-powered blender, followed by the fruit. Blend until smooth. Makes about 32 oz.

# berry green smoothie

## ingredients

- ○ ½ C Frozen Blueberries
- ○ ½ C Frozen Raspberries
- ○ ½ C Frozen Strawberries
- ○ 1 Banana
- ○ 2 C Water
- ○ 1 Large Handful of Spinach

## prepare

Put water and spinach in a Vitamix or other high-powered blender, followed by the fruit. Blend until smooth. Makes about 32 oz.

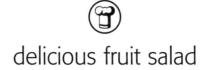

# delicious fruit salad

## ingredients

- ○ 1 Pint Blueberries
- ○ 1 Pint Raspberries
- ○ 2 C Diced Strawberries
- ○ 1 Diced Mango
- ○ 1 Diced Peach

## prepare

Mix in a bowl.

## notes

This recipe is so good that people never believe that it only has fruit in it—they insist it must have added sugar or syrup, but it doesn't!

# scrumptuous couscous

## ingredients

- ○ 6 Chopped Green Onions
- ○ 1 Diced Carrot
- ○ ½ C Diced Tomato
- ○ ½ C Raisins
- ○ 2 C Uncooked Whole Wheat Couscous
- ○ 1½ C Vegetable Broth
- ○ 1 C Apple Juice
- ○ 2-3 t Curry Powder
- ○ Almonds

## prepare

Sauté green onions, carrot and tomato in water, about 5 minutes. Add raisins for one more minute. Add the couscous, broth, apple juice, curry powder, and salt. Bring to a boil, cover, then remove from heat. Let stand about 5 minutes, until the liquid is absorbed. Stir in almonds.

# light and tasty quinoa

## ingredients

- O 1 C diced Onion
- O 2-3 Cloves Garlic
- O ½ t Red Pepper Flakes
- O 1 t Cumin
- O 1 C Quinoa
- O 2 Cans Diced Tomatoes, Drained, Juice Reserved
- O 1½ C Vegetable Broth
- O 1 Can No-Salt Black Beans
- O 1 T Lime Juice
- O 2 T Chopped Cilantro

## prepare

Sauté onion, cumin, garlic and pepper flakes about 3-5 minutes. Add quinoa, reserved tomato juice, and broth. Cover and cook until the quinoa is tender and most of the liquid has been absorbed - about 10 minutes. Add tomatoes, black beans, corn and lime juice. Stir until heated through, about 3 minutes. Sprinkle with cilantro.

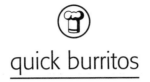

# quick burritos

## ingredients

- ○ Burrito Wrappers (the corn ones are great!)
- ○ 1 Package Ground Tofu, Mexican Flavored
- ○ Vegan, Low-Fat Refried Beans
- ○ Shredded Lettuce
- ○ Diced Tomatoes
- ○ Salsa and/or Hot Sauce
- ○ Onions (optional)
- ○ Cilantro (optional)

## prepare

Heat ground tofu in a skillet with about half a cup of water until warm (about 5 minutes.) Heat refried beans in a microwave. Assemble ingredients in a warm burrito wrapper as desired.

# incredible veggie ceviche

## ingredients

- ○ ½ Red Onion, diced
- ○ 3 Tomatoes, diced
- ○ 1 Red Pepper, diced
- ○ 1 Green Pepper, diced
- ○ 1 C Corn
- ○ 2 Cans Black Beans (or pinto, or a mix)
- ○ 1 Avocado, diced
- ○ 8 Sprigs Cilantro, diced
- ○ 3 T Red Wine Vinegar
- ○ Dash of Cayenne Pepper
- ○ Juice of one Lemon
- ○ Dash of Tabasco Sauce

## prepare

Mix all ingredients in a big bowl and serve!

## notes

This is one of my all-time favorite recipes. I never make it without someone asking for a copy!

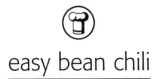

# easy bean chili

## ingredients

- ○ 1 Large Onion, chopped
- ○ 1/3 C Celery, chopped
- ○ 2 Garlic Cloves, minced
- ○ 1 Package Ground Tofu, Original Flavor (optional)
- ○ 1 6 oz Can Tomato Paste
- ○ 1 14.5 oz Can Plum Tomatoes, drained and chopped
- ○ 2 T Chili Powder
- ○ ½ t Ground Cumin
- ○ 2 C Water
- ○ 1 T Lemon Juice
- ○ 2 15 oz Cans Black Beans, drained and rinsed

## prepare

In a large saucepan, heat onion, celery, garlic and ground tofu in a small amount of water on the stove, about 5 minutes. Add the tomato paste, tomatoes, chili powder, cumin and water. Simmer for 30 minutes, adding more water if needed. Add the lemon juice and beans, and simmer for another 15 minutes, adding water if needed. When serving, top with a tablespoon of cilantro pesto (next page.) As my nephew, Barrett, would say, "Deeeeeee-licious!"

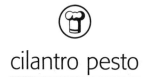

# cilantro pesto

## ingredients

- O 1 C Tightly Packed Cilantro Leaves
- O ¼ C Raw Almonds
- O 2 Large Garlic Cloves
- O ½ t Salt
- O ¼ C Olive Oil

## prepare

Combine in a food processor until smooth. Serve one tablespoon of pesto on top of chili. Enjoy!

## notes

This pesto is fantastic on top of chili. Just adding it can help you win a chili cook-off!

# super easy pizza

## ingredients

- ○ Pizza Crust
- ○ Pizza Sauce
- ○ Capers
- ○ Mushrooms
- ○ Sun-Dried Tomatoes
- ○ Artichoke Hearts
- ○ Kalamata Olives
- ○ Pine Nuts
- ○ Broccoli Florets, cut very small

## prepare

Spread pizza sauce over crust. Top with as many toppings as you'd like. The ones listed here are just a suggestion. Use whatever veggies you have that look good to you. Corn is great, and I love adding avocado after the pizza comes out of the oven! Cook according to the pizza crust package instructions, usually about 15 minutes. Enjoy!

## notes

Natural food stores usually carry vegan pizza crusts in their frozen foods section.

# sarah's favorite lima bean soup

## ingredients

- ○ 3 C Dry Lima Beans
- ○ 1 C Chopped Onion
- ○ 6 C Hot Water
- ○ 3 Celery Ribs, sliced into small pieces
- ○ 1 T Dried Rosemary
- ○ 1 T Dried Sage
- ○ Balsamic Vinegar
- ○ Black Pepper

## prepare

Soak beans overnight in plenty of water and rinse. Put all ingredients except vinegar into a large soup pot and cook over low-medium heat until the beans are tender. Watch beans in case they foam and overflow—keep the lid off the pot to help reduce this risk. When beans are tender, use a potato masher to mash some of the beans up and make the soup a bit creamier. Add balsamic vinegar and black pepper to taste. You can add salt on your individual serving if necessary. When you haven't had meat for a long time, this soup will taste surprisingly like it has turkey in it!

# hearty african bean stew

## ingredients

- ○ 3 C 12 Bean Mix, soaked overnight in plenty of water
- ○ 4 t Garlic, minced
- ○ 4 C Coarsely Chopped Onions
- ○ 10 C Hot Water
- ○ 4 Large Carrots, sliced into small pieces
- ○ 3 T Ground Coriander Seeds
- ○ 5 t Dried Mint
- ○ 4 t Ground Cumin Seeds
- ○ 1 T Ground Caraway Seeds
- ○ ½ Crushed Red Pepper Flakes
- ○ 4 T Tomato Paste
- ○ 5 T Balsamic Vinegar

## prepare

Soak beans overnight and rinse. Cook garlic and onions in a small amount of water for about 1 minute. Add all ingredients except tomato paste and vinegar. Cook until beans are tender. (About 2 hours or so—check frequently.) Add tomato paste and balsamic vinegar. Serve with whole wheat crusty bread. Very hearty, and delicious!

# indian potato and pea curry

## ingredients

- ○ 1 Small Onion, sliced
- ○ 2 Medium Potatoes, cut into bite-sized pieces
- ○ 2 T Minced Ginger
- ○ 3 Cloves Garlic
- ○ 1 T Curry Powder
- ○ 1 tsp Ground Cumin
- ○ 1 tsp Turmeric
- ○ 2 C Vegetable Broth
- ○ ½ C Light Coconut Milk
- ○ 1 Medium Head Cauliflower, cut into florets
- ○ 2 Zucchini, sliced into small round pieces
- ○ 1 C Frozen Peas
- ○ 3 T Chopped Cilantro

## prepare

Sauté onion in water, about 3 minutes. Add potatoes, ginger, garlic, curry powder, cumin and turmeric. Cook 3 minutes. Add broth and coconut milk. Bring to a boil, reduce heat, cover and simmer for 10 minutes. Add cauliflower and zucchini and cook another 10 minutes, uncovered. Stir in peas and cilantro. Yum!

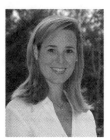

## SARAH TAYLOR, MBA

Sarah Taylor has been a vegan since 2002 when she read *Diet for a New America* by John Robbins. Both the philosophy and the science supporting a vegan diet convinced her to go vegan, and she has never looked back.

In 2006, Sarah started a company called "The Vegan Next Door," in an effort to spread the word about the vegan diet. She is now a motivational speaker, trainer and author.

In her personal time, Sarah serves on the Board of Directors at Washington Women's Employment and Education, enjoys playing competitive tennis, scuba diving, reading and adventure traveling. She is happily married and lives in Gig Harbor, WA with her husband and many pets.

# help us spread the word!

Have you become a vegan?
We would love to post your story, photo(s) and testimonials on our growing website and in our marketing materials!

Please send general correspondence to:
**info@TheVeganNextDoor.com**

You can contact Sarah Taylor at:
**Sarah@TheVeganNextDoor.com**

And don't forget to visit our website!
**www.TheVeganNextDoor.com**